Not Now . . . I'm Having a No Hair Day handles grave subject matter with sensitivity and warmth. And, who could not smile at the wonderful illustrations by Jack Lindstrom.

Jim Davis
cartoonist and creator of Garfield™

Not Now . . . I'm Having a No Hair Day should be a daily companion of anyone who has been touched by cancer. Readers will cherish the laughter and tears that have gone into this book.

Burton S. Schwartz, M.D.
Medical oncologist

We can't laugh off the seriousness of cancer—but we can learn to turn on an inner chemistry that supplements conventional cancer treatment. *Not Now . . . I'm Having a No Hair Day* will help individuals unlock their individual body-mind pharmacy to fulfill a physiological prescription that can add days to life and life to days.

Dale L. Anderson, M.D.
President, J'ARM, Inc.

To Kay,

Celebrate 5 years!
Don't forget to laugh!

Christine Clifford

Not now...
I'm having a

No Hair
Day

**CHRISTINE
CLIFFORD**

Illustrations by
JACK LINDSTROM

*Humor & Healing
for People with Cancer*

Pfeifer-Hamilton Publishers
Duluth, Minnesota

Pfeifer-Hamilton Publishers
210 West Michigan
Duluth, MN 55802

Not Now . . . I'm Having a No Hair Day

Printed in the United States of America
10 9 8 7 6 5 4 3

Editorial Director: Susan Gustafson
Graphic Design: Joy Morgan Dey

Library of Congress Cataloging in Publication Data
Clifford, Christine, 1954–
   Not now . . . I'm having a no hair day / written by Christine Clifford
 ; illustrations by Jack Lindstrom.
      112 p. 15 cm.
   ISBN 1-57025-120-7
   1. Cancer—Psychosomatic aspects. 2. Cancer—Humor.   I. Title.
RC262.C526   1996
362.1 ' 96994—dc20   96—10027
                         CIP

Dedication

To my mother and to all those everywhere
whose lives have been touched by cancer

Foreword

Tom Weiskopf, Senior PGA Tour player

Chris and my wife, Jeanne, have both overcome breast cancer, having gone through surgery, chemo, and radiation. These beautiful ladies did this with determination, a positive attitude, and a profound respect for the most important reason God created us, life itself.

Both women love living life and its challenges to their fullest—and always with a sense of humor. Reading Chris's book brought back memories of my feelings during the past year. With humor and insight, Chris presents the reality of what may happen to the cancer patient and to family and friends.

If a friend or family member has cancer, support them with all your love, and, as Chris reminds us, use laughter to bring happiness back into their lives.

Chris Clifford and Jeanne Weiskopf, through their determination, have made me a stronger person. Oh, by the way, ladies, have you noticed? I've been having bad hair days for a lot longer than both of you put together.

Acknowledgments

I would like to thank the following individuals for helping make *Not Now . . . I'm Having a No Hair Day* a reality:

My dear friend Jeanne Weiskopf, her husband, Tom, and their daughter, Heidi, for paving the way and lending a good ear; my editor, Susan Gustafson, and Pfeifer-Hamilton for taking a chance; my illustrator, Jack Lindstrom, for capturing the essence of my being.

My sister, Pam Meyer, for always being there for me; my parents-in-law, John and Bette Clifford, for accepting me as the daughter they never had but always wanted; and my stepmother, Stephanie Meyer, for her words of encouragement.

My dear friends Whitney and Nancy Peyton and Bill and Barb Winchell for helping me find something to focus on.

Dr. James Gaviser for leading me to a superior team of medical professionals: Dr. Margit L. Bretzke; the staff at Minnesota Oncology

Hematology, including Dr. Burton Schwartz and Ann Nelson; Dr. Tae Kim and the technicians at Abbott Northwestern Hospital.

My employers, Bob Brown and Bill Bartels, for telling me, "You can do it!"

Joan Wernick for being a good listener.

The thousands of friends, acquaintances, associates, and strangers who believed in me and offered daily words of encouragement. Special thanks to: my neighbors, Molly Gill-Ramczyk, Twila Donley, Joan and Stuart Brooks, Pat Miles, JohnMichael, James Stirratt, Craig Moen, Gail See, Carol Britton, Martha Edgar, Dr. Dale Anderson, Paula Bergs, Jeff Evans, and Nancy Selleck.

But most of all, I would like to thank my loving husband, John, with whom I celebrated twenty years of marriage on a chemotherapy day, and my sons, Tim and Brooks, for their love, support, friendship, and sense of humor.

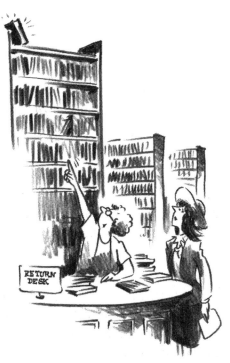

"HUMOROUS BOOKS ON CANCER?...SURE,
RIGHT UP THERE ON THAT TOP SHELF."

Introduction

I cannot pinpoint the exact moment in time when humor became a purposeful part of my treatment for breast cancer. I do know I had an "a-hah!" moment that has altered my life profoundly.

Days, weeks, and months passed as I endured surgery, completed radiation treatment, and plugged on through chemotherapy. Not a day went by that I didn't receive cards, calls, flowers, or meals from family, friends, neighbors, and business associates. But with all the loving gestures of friendship and support, somehow I felt there was something missing.

Then it occurred to me. Not once in six months had anyone brought or sent me anything that made me laugh. I had a three-foot pile of books on the floor of my closet that I never read. They were either too medical, too analytical, or they were self-help books that didn't seem to provide any answers as I threw up after chemotherapy or worried about sunburn on my recently bald head.

Just once, I thought, I wish someone would bring me something to make me laugh. I had cried so many tears the well was dry. I needed the tonic and release of laughter. I needed something to fill me back up.

Once I understood what I needed, I found humor around me everywhere. Real-life humor was just begging to be picked up and shared. Kids—and grown-ups—really do say the darndest things! And life with cancer has a great many funny moments, as well as a lot of serious ones.

People are the only creatures on earth who can laugh. To laugh is to rejoice in being alive. Laughter flings open the shutters and lets the sunshine in. A shared gift of laughter is a priceless gift to the spirit. And it's a great poke in the eye to the adversary that cancer patients are struggling every day to beat.

This book is dedicated to everyone who has ever known the disease we call cancer. Whether you're a cancer survivor, a family member of an affected loved one, a friend, or a patient, I hope this book will bring laughter into your life.

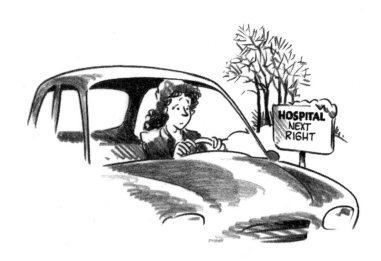

Nothing to laugh about

There is nothing humorous
about getting
a diagnosis of cancer.

The day it happened to me will remain etched in my memory forever . . .

I had been having annual mammograms since I was thirty years old because of my mother's early death at age forty-two from breast cancer. Every year the mammograms were a frightening experience for me. Would the test reveal something this time? Sometimes I actually fainted from the anxiety.

Until I was thirty-five, I resisted doing self-exams of my breasts for the same reason. What if I found a lump? Would I wither and die like my mother did?

By the end of the year I turned forty, everything in my life was going beautifully. My husband, John, and I were approaching our twentieth wedding anniversary. We had two beautiful, active boys, Tim, eleven, and Brooks, eight. I was just completing the most successful year of my career as senior vice president of a large international marketing company. And John and I were a month away from submitting an offer on the house of our dreams. I was on top of the world.

Then, on November 9th, my life came to a screeching halt.

I was doing a breast self exam when I felt something small and unusual in my right breast. I called a leading hospital in Minneapolis and explained, "I'm a forty-year-old woman whose mother died of breast cancer. I've found a lump in my breast." They said they'd see me that day. As I drove to the hospital, my throat in a knot, all I could think was, "This is how it all begins."

I was examined by two doctors. Neither of them felt the lump. They said that in this routine exam they didn't detect anything out of the ordinary. I showed each of them where I'd felt something suspicious, and they both acknowledged that "something" seemed to be there. I was given a mammogram, just two months before my annual exam had been scheduled. Nothing showed up on the films. At that point the doctors told me I probably had nothing to worry about. My lump was in the least likely place in the breast for cancer ("less than 10 percent likelihood," they said). It hurt, and I was told that cancer doesn't hurt. Besides, it felt soft. Cancer, they said, feels like a marble or a pea. They said I probably had a cyst or a blood clot. I should go home, leave it alone, and come back in thirty days.

I waited for twenty-five days and cheated every day—I couldn't keep my fingers off that lump! When I felt it was definitely getting bigger, I decided to go to my gynecologist for a second opinion. He had delivered my two sons, he knew my family history, he worked for a breast cancer detection clinic, and he was one of only a handful of gynecologists in the state who performed breast cancer surgery. Though the lump was more pronounced, he agreed with the original diagnosis. He looked at me reassuringly and said, "Don't lose any sleep over this, Chris. You don't have cancer."

"But I *am* losing sleep over it. I'm a wreck," I protested. Just to be safe, my doctor decided to perform a needle biopsy. If fluid came out, he explained, we'd know for sure it was a cyst.

I could hardly look as what seemed like a twelve-inch needle was shoved deep into my breast. To my watchful eyes, the doctor appeared concerned when blood came out rather than the liquid we were hoping for. "It's probably a dried blood clot," he said. "You'll have to wait until Monday to get the results. We have to send the sample to California for a reading."

That was the longest weekend of my life.

Monday was the beginning of Christmas week. It was also my youngest son's, birthday, and I'd planned a dinner party that evening to celebrate. I went to work at half past eight as usual, and attended a staff meeting from nine until noon. When I got out of the meeting and received a message to call my doctor, I felt the blood leave my face. The sounds of people talking in my office were drowned out by the ringing in my ears.

I put in the call to the doctor's office. The answering service told me they'd been waiting for my call, and would put me right through. As usual, his nurse answered the phone. I heard her ask my doctor where he wanted to take the call. "I'll take it in 3B," he replied.

"Chris, I'm shocked at what I have to tell you. You tested positive for cancer."

I fell to the floor of my office and didn't hear another word he said . . .

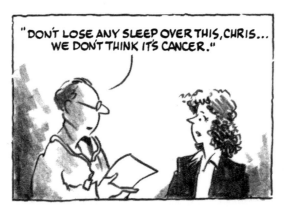

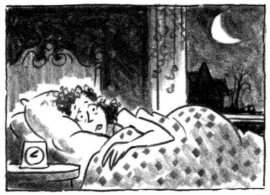

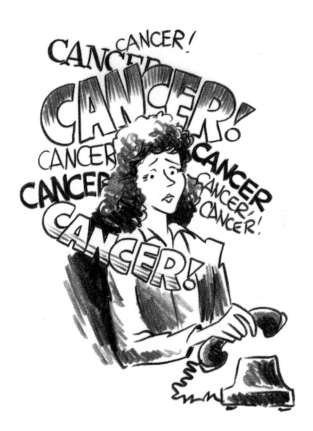

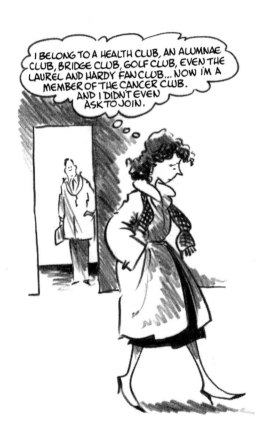

22

Now what?

After I revived,
I called my husband.

"John, please meet me at home."

"What's wrong?" he said, responding to my unusual request and to something he could hear in my voice.

"I have cancer."

After all those years of anxiety, there it was—cancer.

I don't know how I drove home, but John was waiting for me when I walked through the door. We hugged for a long time, me sobbing in his arms. From that moment on, John took control of the situation.

We immediately went to see my gynecologist. He told us he could do the necessary surgery on Tuesday or Wednesday of that week at the local community hospital where he practiced, or I could wait until after the holidays. One more week wouldn't make any difference, he said. Even though I tried to concentrate, I couldn't seem to hear a word he said as he explained the pros and cons of mastectomies versus lumpectomies, reconstructive surgery, chemotherapy, and radiation.

I decided to have the surgery after Christmas so as not to spoil the holidays for the boys. We drove home, threw the dinner party, celebrated Brooks's birthday, and didn't tell a soul. When the last guest had left the house, I broke down and cried for the next three days without stopping.

By that time we had informed my sister, my in-laws, my two best friends, and the president of my corporation. With only three days left before Christmas, I decided I needed to take charge and investigate the options in front of me.

I contacted the only other two doctors involved in my life—my family internist and my dermatologist—and asked them for referrals to a plastic surgeon. Since I only had a needle biopsy, I wouldn't know when I went into surgery whether the operation was going to be a mastectomy or a lumpectomy. Amazingly, both doctors recommended the same person. It was now the Wednesday before Christmas, but when I called him, he told me he could see me that very day.

I can only vaguely recall our conversation about reconstructive surgery. I remember words like *modified, radical, implants,* and *subcutaneous,* but I was still in a state of denial, and it was hard to take it all in. I do clearly recall when he put his hands on my shoulders, looked me squarely in the eye and said, "Chris, if I can make one recommendation, please allow me to refer you to a general surgeon who specializes in breast cancer surgery. You go home, and I'll make the necessary appointments."

I recontacted my gynecologist and asked if he also could arrange some referrals. "Chris, it's just a couple of days before Christmas," he said. "I seriously doubt if you'll be able to see anybody. But if you're willing to try, here are some phone numbers."

Of course, when I tried to call the doctors he'd referred me to it was like trying to get in touch with the Pope! No one would see me until after the holidays, and they seemed frustratingly unco-operative. The plastic surgeon, however, had more success. By six o'clock the same day he was able to schedule appointments with a general surgeon, a top oncologist, and a radiologist—all on the Thursday and Friday before Christmas.

My first appointment on Thursday was with the oncologist, a warm and gentle man who spent almost two hours with John and me. When I explained my symptoms to him, his response was to take a routine urinalysis and to schedule me for a complete bone scan during the next week. Well aware that I was only "shopping" for doctors at this point, he explained that since these were neces-sary procedures that would have to be completed prior to my sur-gery he would be glad to forward the results of the bone scan to whichever doctors I chose. I remember asking myself and John why my gynecologist hadn't explained that to me when I'd talked to him.

That afternoon I met with the head of radiology at the same prestigious hospital I'd gone to the day I found my lump. He was a kind and caring doctor who carefully explained the radia-tion procedure, introduced me to the staff, and gave me a tour of the hospital facilities. I went home feeling much more knowledge-able and secure about what lay ahead of me.

On Friday I met with the general surgeon. She was a woman, close to my age. She also took the time necessary to make me feel as comfortable as possible.

That night I struggled with the pros and cons of using my own gynecologist, whom I had known for thirteen years, or putting my life in the hands of strangers.

On Christmas Day the phone rang at three in the afternoon. It was the woman surgeon. "How are you holding up, Chris?" she inquired. "And how are your children taking the news?" I was deeply touched by her concern. I told her we would be telling them the next day.

By Christmas night I had made my decisions. I chose the woman surgeon and the oncologist and radiologist I'd consulted with. I also decided to continue my treatment at the hospital where I had first gone, despite the errant diagnosis I'd originally received. All the doctors I'd chosen, a completely different group than the ones who had originally examined me, practiced at the hospital; it was highly reputable; and I'd developed a strong degree of comfort and confidence through the visits and tours I'd made in the past few days.

The day after Christmas, John and I called the two boys into the family room, and John told them we needed to have a family chat.

"Didn't we have a nice Christmas?" he said, surveying the toys and candy strewn all over the house.

"Yes!" they squealed.

"Aren't we a lucky family?" he asked.

"Yes," they both nodded.

"Well, sometimes, along with the good things in life, come some bad things," John began.

"Thank you for sharing that with us, Dad," Brooks quipped. John and I looked at each other and burst into laughter.

Then, "Your mom has a disease called cancer," John told them. "She will be going to the hospital and will have to have several treatments over the next few months. The treatments will make her very sick, and she may lose her hair."

"Cool!" Tim exclaimed. "Will you look like Captain Jean-Luc Picard on Star Trek?"

In the next few hours the boys both came to me, individually, and asked me the question I didn't want to hear. "Mom, will you die?" I hugged them as tightly as I could and assured them I wasn't ready to leave this earth.

My sister Pam called to say she would be there for my surgery. She flew in from New York the night before.

The surgery was scheduled for seven o'clock on the morning of New Year's Eve.

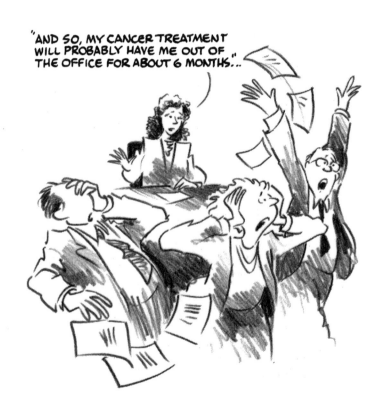

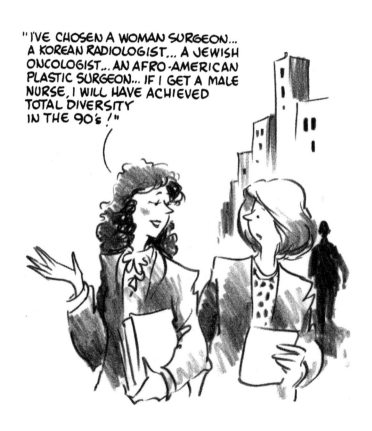

31

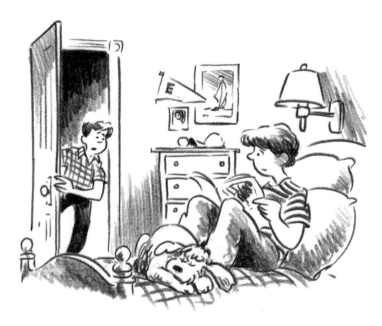

"HEY, TIM...MOM AND DAD WANT TO DISCUSS SOMETHING IMPORTANT WITH US...YOU DON'T SUPPOSE THE GERBIL GOT LOOSE AGAIN, DO YOU?"

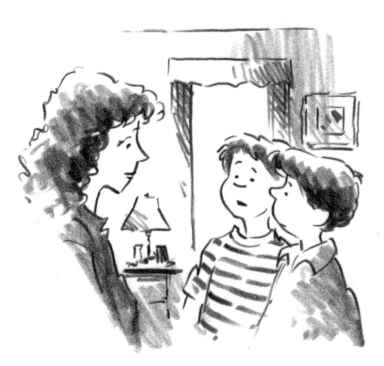

"MOM...IS THIS BREAST CANCER THING HEREDITARY?"

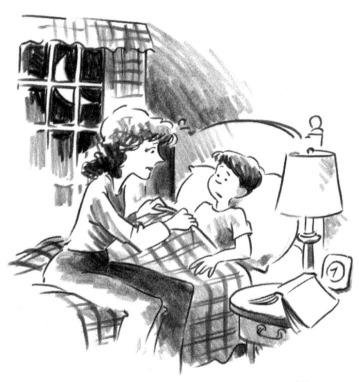

"MOM...WHEN CAN I STOP WORRYING?"

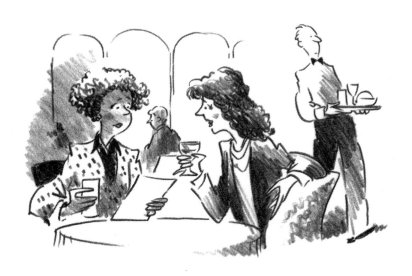

"YES, THE DOCTOR DID SAY 'NO ALCOHOL 48 HOURS BEFORE
CANCER SURGERY'... SO WHAT'S IT GOING TO DO, KILL ME?"

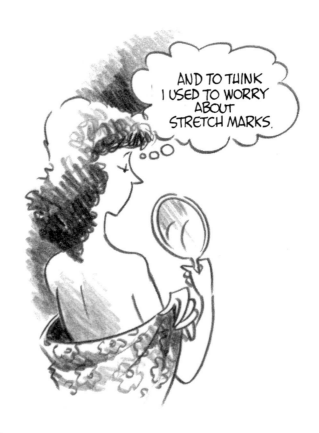

Welcome to the New Year!

I could never begin
to describe the fear I felt
going into surgery.

I had always taken great pride in my girlish figure and worked hard to maintain my shape as the years passed. In the days before the operation, I would often catch myself pausing in front of a mirror to look at my body and wonder what it would be like after surgery.

The night before my operation, I carefully took out the dress I had planned to wear to a big party on New Year's Eve. It was a beautiful red dress, low cut to reveal my cleavage. I slowly put it on to remember myself that way for one last time.

That evening I cried for hours, and John held me in his arms until

I dozed off to sleep. We had to be at the hospital at five in the morning, and I don't think I got more than an hour or two of sleep.

When we arrived at the hospital, my minister was there to greet us. As I was prepped and readied for surgery, I still couldn't contain my tears. The last thing I remember was the plastic surgeon saying to the anesthesiologist, "Let's put her out."

When I awoke, the first face I saw was that of my plastic surgeon. Before panic could overwhelm me, he quickly assured me they'd been able to save my breast, but that the lump had been very deep. "We've never seen anything quite like it," he said. "It was down on the chest muscle wall, which is why it didn't show up on the mammogram. And that also explains why it hurt."

He told me I'd had a lumpectomy and an axillary lymph node dissection, and that they'd also removed the lining of the chest wall muscle. He explained that they couldn't remove any of the chest muscle, since it is necessary for arm movement. The traditional treatment of muscle cancer would be chemotherapy and radiation.

That evening a stream of friends and family stopped by the hospital on their way to various New Year's Eve festivities. My sister

Pam and John stayed with me until midnight to welcome in the New Year. And the children along with their grandparents visited for a few short hours as well. I passed the next days taking calls from well-wishers and learning more about the upcoming treatment and recovery process from hospital staff, nurses, volunteers, and other patients. I worried about things at the office, but was quickly assured by my staff and employer that everything at work was under control.

Four days later the pathology report came back. On the Nottingham scale which grades tumors from one to three, with three being the most severe, my tumor had been a grade three. It was a rapidly dividing tumor (with what's called a "brisk mitotic rate"), and the doctors' concern was with the cancer that was still in my chest muscle. My thirteen lymph nodes, which had been removed, were clear of cancer cells.

Because of my age, my family history, the size of the tumor, and where it was located, the doctors decided on an aggressive treatment plan that included doing both chemotherapy and radiation at the same time. They told me they believed that my cancer had been developing for almost three years.

When it was time to leave the hospital, it was quite a challenge to load the car with all the flowers and gifts that had poured into the hospital during my stay. I felt relieved to be leaving the hospital for the warmth and comfort of my own home and bed, but a wave of anxiety came over me as the nurse rolled me out the doors in the customary wheelchair.

The chemo adventure was about to begin.

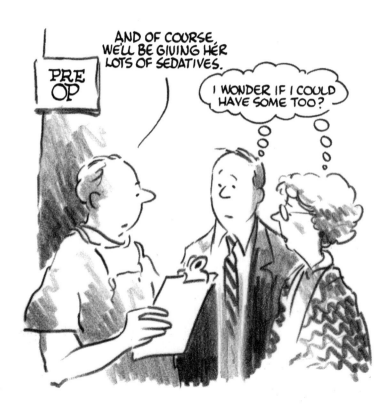

41

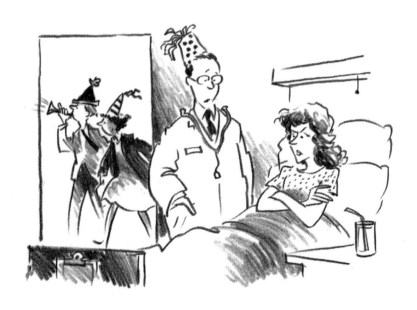

"SORRY ABOUT THE TIMING OF YOUR SURGERY, CHRIS... NEW YEAR'S EVE PROBABLY WOULD'NT HAVE BEEN YOUR FIRST CHOICE."

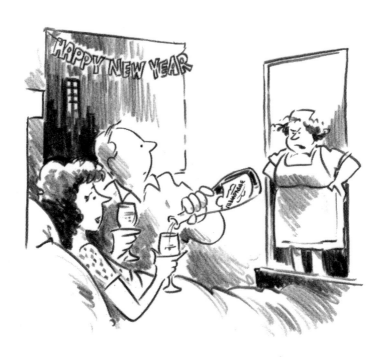

"DEMEROL AND ALCOHOL?...DON'T EVEN THINK ABOUT IT!"

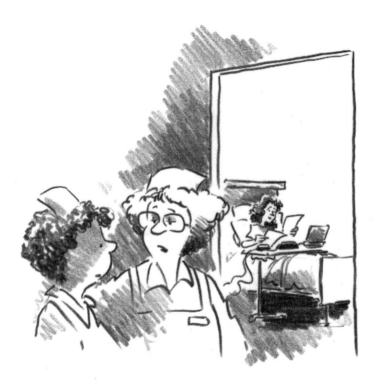

"14B BROUGHT HER LAPTOP, FAX MACHINE, PRINTER AND CELLULAR TELEPHONE WITH HER... SHE MUST BE OUT OF 'SICK' DAYS."

44

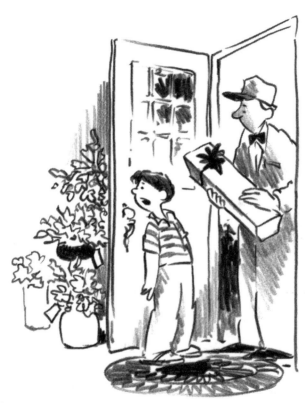

"MOM... MORE FLOWERS FOR YOUR BREAST!"

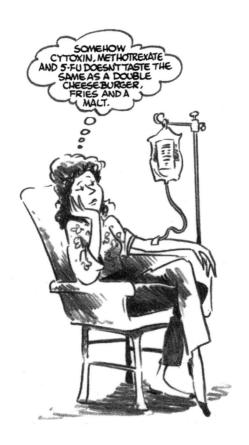

One day at a time

Why don't they just take me outside and shoot me?

That was my thought after John and I attended a special chemo-therapy class, where we learned about all the side effects I was about to experience. I was going to lose my hair, feel sick, have mouth sores, and go through menopause.

The chemotherapy would be administered for two weeks in a row, then I'd be off it for two weeks, then back on for another two. It was to alternate like that for six months. After one month of chemotherapy, my radiation treatments would begin as well.

I knew that of all the side effects I was about to experience, losing my hair would be the most traumatic. I can actually remember wondering if I would be able to hear the sound of my hair falling out.

Molly, one of my best friends, made arrangements with John, unbeknownst to me, to take me to a wig salon that specialized in serving cancer patients. It was intimidating to walk into the shop, but the owner was a compassionate and friendly woman named Twila. She quickly made me feel at home, whisked me into a private salon where we had complete privacy, and we instantly became friends for life.

Of course, at this point I had a complete head of thick, curly hair—my pride and joy. Twila explained that this was an advantage, as she could design a hairpiece to look exactly like my own hair. Molly and I laughed until we cried as I tried on different colors, styles, lengths, and textures. We finally settled on a beautiful, natural hairpiece that would be styled just like my own hair. The wig, I was told, would be ready to pick up whenever I needed it.

I learned in chemotherapy class that when the treatment started, I would be given three chemotherapy drugs: Methotrexate, Cytoxan, and 5-FU; a steroid to increase appetite and improve my energy level; and a powerful drug to prevent nausea and vomiting.

Each treatment took approximately three hours, but because I also needed various kinds of blood tests and an appointment with the doctor, I'd be at the clinic for four to five hours twice each month.

From the sound of things, I knew chemotherapy would be a lot to deal with, and it was. I decided to take things one day at a time, which proved to be a good approach. Some days and some moments were tougher than others.

The drugs I took to combat nausea were extremely effective. I combined them with a strong "mind over matter" attitude and resolved to get through the chemo as best I could. The most difficult part for me was dealing with a lifelong phobia about needles that caused me to faint two or three times in the following months as the nurses connected me to the IV.

During the procedure itself, I read, watched TV, or talked to other patients, John, or the staff at the clinic. Some days the treatment seemed to take an eternity, and other times I was amazed at how quickly the time flew by.

The effects of the chemotherapy didn't really hit me until six or eight hours later. Then I took a few more antinausea pills, crawled into bed, and hoped for the best.

My hair began to fall out slowly, first in patches after my third or fourth treatment and finally in handfuls that clogged the shower drain and left me staring at the floor in amazement. I phoned Twila, picked up my wig, bought a few additional hairpieces, and decided that hats were the wave of the future.

Throughout my treatments, in spite of all the changes that were taking place in my life, I never felt that I was alone. John, the boys, my friends and family, coworkers, and acquaintances by the score were with me every step of the way. Day by day, the weeks passed as our family adjusted to living with the routine and the effects of chemotherapy.

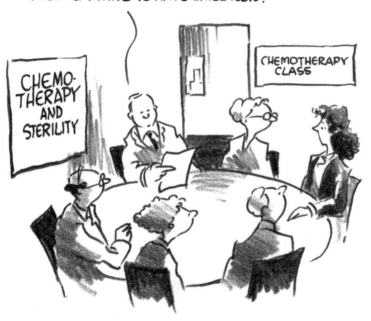

51

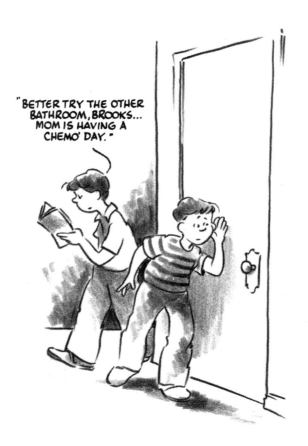

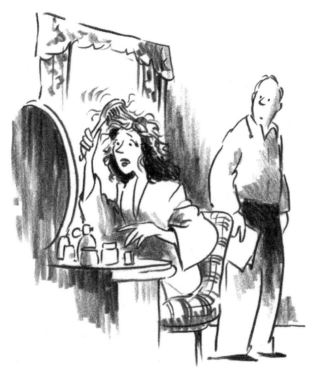

"TURN UP THE RADIO WILL YOU, SWEETHEART... LOUD ENOUGH TO COVER THE SOUND OF MY HAIR FALLING OUT, ...PLEASE."

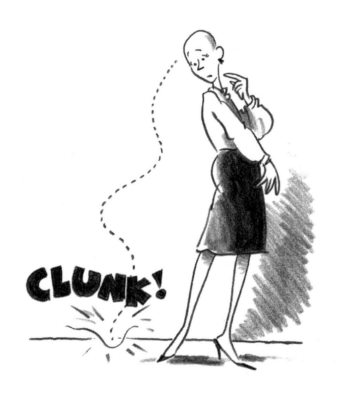

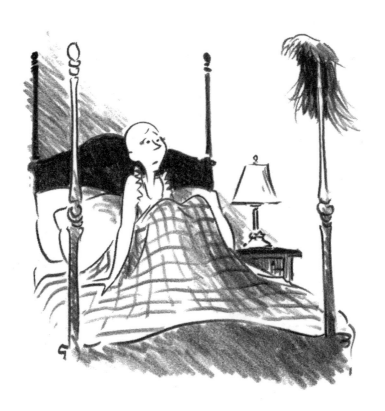

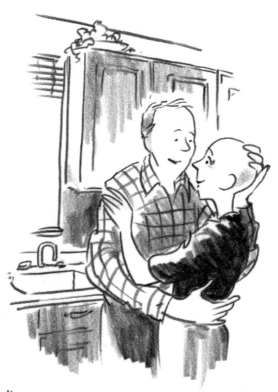

"LOOK AT IT THIS WAY, HONEY... THERE'S MORE OF YOU TO KISS."

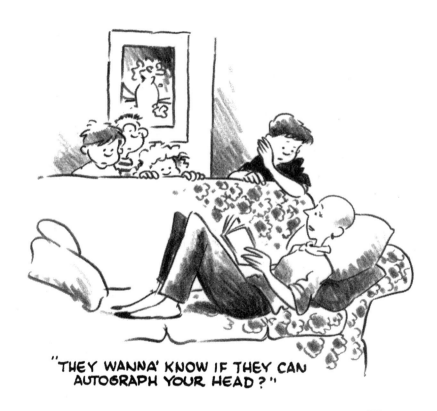

"THEY WANNA' KNOW IF THEY CAN AUTOGRAPH YOUR HEAD?"

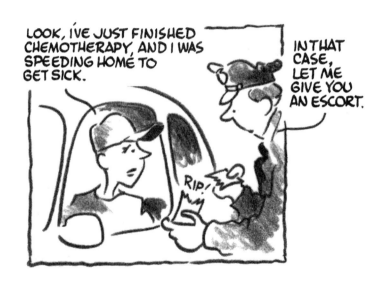

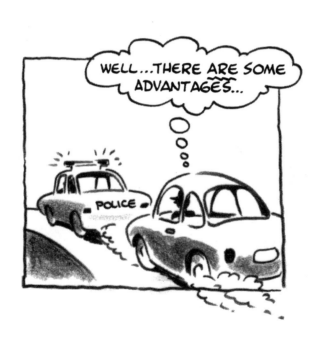

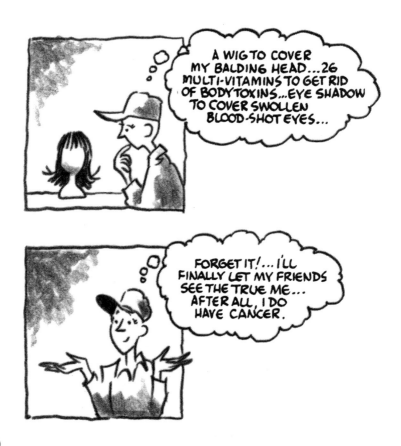

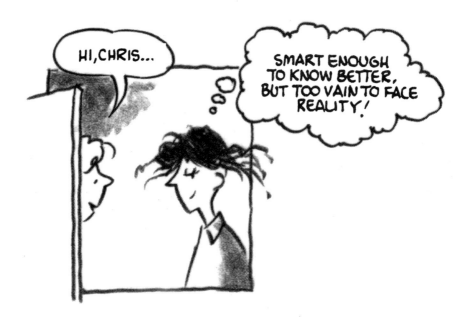

61

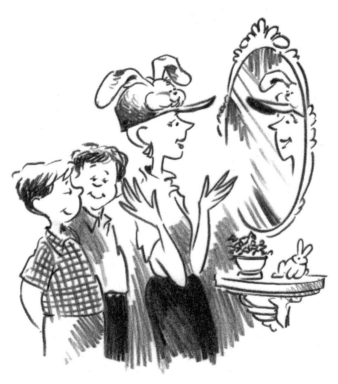

"OH, TIMMY...BROOKS! IT'S SO ME!"

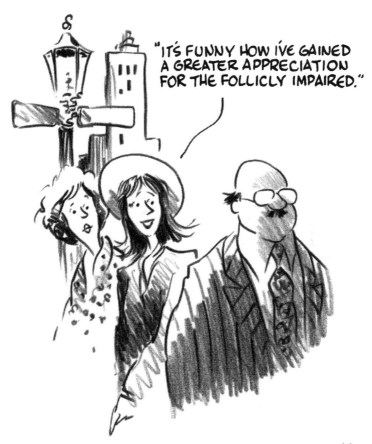

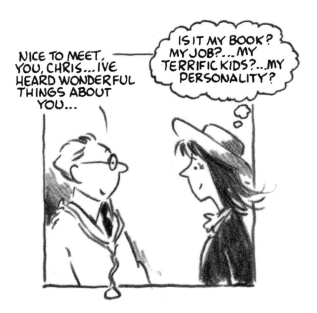

64

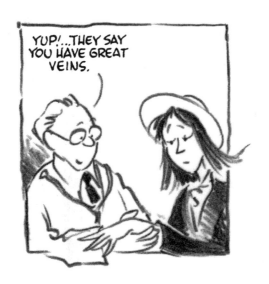

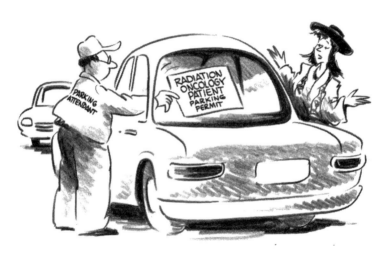

"OH, GREAT... WHY DON'T WE JUST HANG A BANNER ON IT THAT SAYS 'CANCER VICTIM'?"

Therapy two-step: dancing with the "Big Machine"

After a month of chemo alone, it was time to begin radiation.

The "sandwich effect," it was called—one treatment on top of the other.

I made a trip to the hospital for a simulation, or run-through, to get the correct measurements, to have a mold made for my upper body and arms, and to get "marked." To mark the field for radiation dark black "X's" were drawn on various parts of my chest and breasts and covered with tape. I was told it was important that the marks be kept in place for the next several months.

I was also given a sign to put in the window of my car that read:

```
Christine Clifford
Parking Permit
Radiation Therapy
2/23/95—4/28/95
```

I felt as though I had a billboard on top of my car announcing, "Cancer Patient On Board!" I was very self-conscious about my "X's" as well. I had to change the style of clothing I was used to wearing to keep them well-hidden from the general public.

Every morning for thirty-three days I went to the hospital at ten o'clock to get my daily blast of radiation. The major side effects of radiation treatment were extreme exhaustion, tenderness of the breast, and a sunburned appearance of the area being radiated.

The hospital staff and I quickly became fast friends as I paraded bare-chested every day to the big machine. The procedure itself didn't take more than five minutes, but I would lie down on the machine, close my eyes, and take a "quick nap." After several weeks, a group of technicians watching me through a monitor asked what I was thinking about as I lay there with my eyes closed. "You look like you're meditating or thinking deep thoughts," they said. Reflecting on the fast pace of my life at the office and the constant commotion of the children at home, I said honestly, "No, I'm just relishing the total tranquility."

I took my children with me many times to watch the procedure. They baked cookies to bring to the technicians, and they gleefully watched me on the TV screens and talked to me through the voice monitors that were used for staff and patient safety.

From day number one, I began a mental process of counting down the days until radiation would be finished. On the last day of treatment, the staff gave me a graduation certificate, a cake, and a round of hearty congratulations. I showed them my appreciation for their support and patience by taking them all out for dinner one evening. I felt I could never thank them enough for making what could have been a frightening and dismal experience into a "walk in the park" that seemed to be over almost as soon as it began.

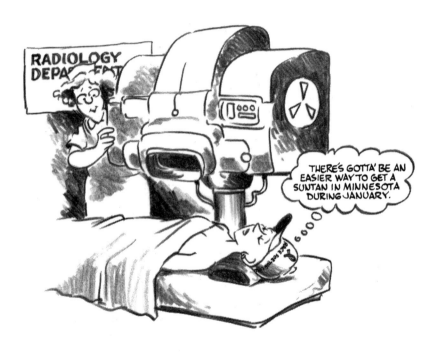

70

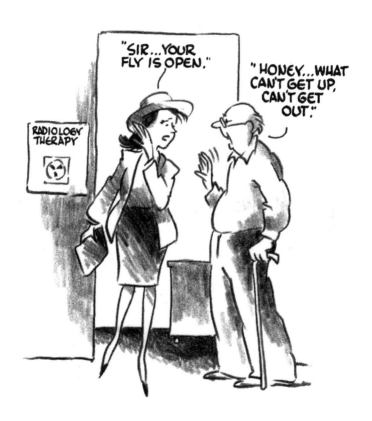

71

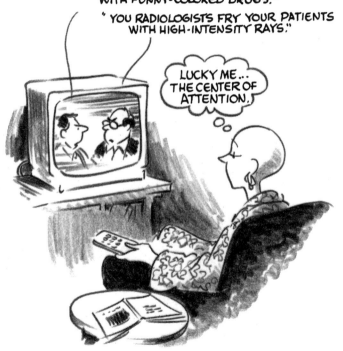

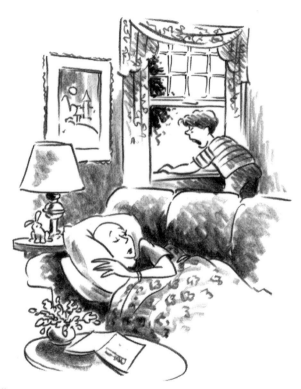

"HEY, RALPH, QUIET OUT THERE...MY MOM'S SLEEPING!"

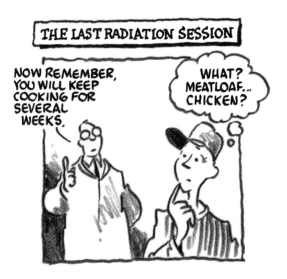

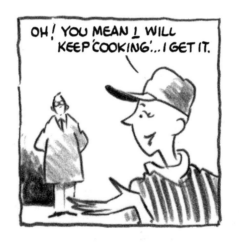

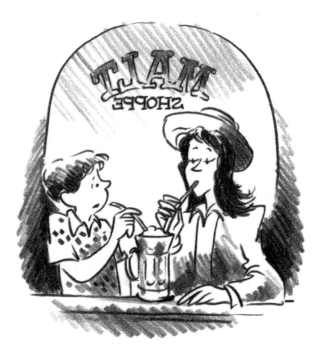

"MOM...IS CANCER CONTAGIOUS?"

Family matters

Cancer gave me one unexpected gift.

I developed a renewed relationship with my family.

As a busy executive, prior to my diagnosis and surgery I was often away on business trips for days, even weeks at a time.

Over the years, John had gradually, willingly, and lovingly taken over most of the major household chores and child-rearing responsibilities: making the lunches, getting the kids off to school, being there when they got home, coaching sports, going to school conferences and after-school activities. I always thought I had a good relationship with my children (the old "quality time," not "quantity time" cliche). It wasn't until I was home every day dealing with cancer that I realized I had not been much more than a ship passing in and out of their lives.

I started sharing activities with the boys that I had often missed because of business commitments. I involved them in my treatments and recovery to relieve their fears and to assure them that I *would* be a survivor!

I didn't want my cancer to disrupt our entire life, so I made a point of getting up every day, putting on my makeup, wig, and hat, and greeting the children with a smile on my face.

John and I celebrated our twentieth wedding anniversary six months into my treatment. We weren't able to take the long-planned trip we had been dreaming of for several years, but as we weathered this storm "in sickness and in health" we realized how lucky we were to have each other as partners.

On the day of our anniversary I had to take a chemotherapy treatment. As I sat in the chair thinking how far I was from the youth, health, and exuberance of twenty years ago, I realized how lucky I was to have my family and to have the opportunity that lay ahead of me to take the time—*make* the time—to enjoy them every day.

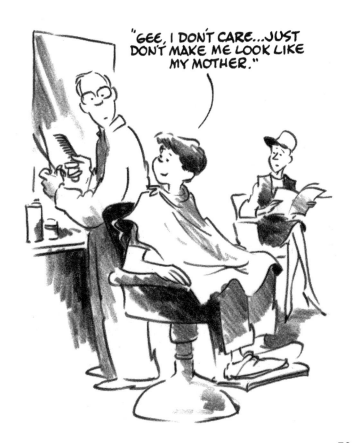

79

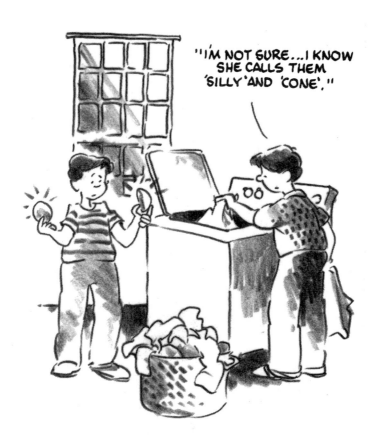

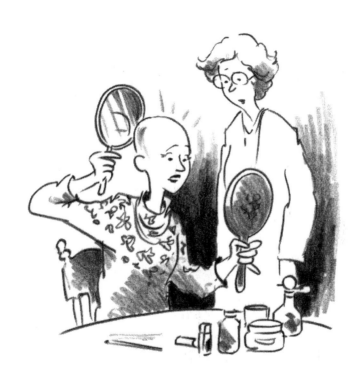

"THEY USED TO ASK, 'HOW'S WORK?' ...OR 'HOW ARE THE KIDS?'
NOW IT'S... 'IS IT GROWING BACK YET?'"

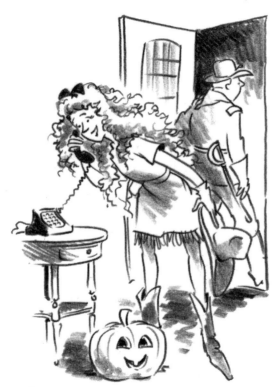

"TO A COSTUME PARTY... I'M GOING AS A PERSON WITH HAIR!"

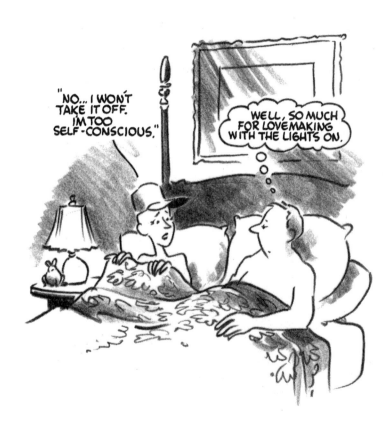

83

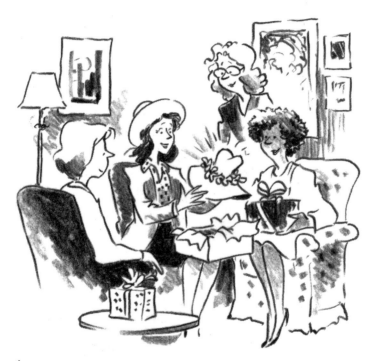

"BRIDAL SHOWERS, YES... BABY SHOWERS, YES... BUT THIS IS MY FIRST CHEMOTHERAPY SHOWER."

That's what friends are for

I have had a rare opportunity indeed.

Within my lifetime, I've had the chance to learn how many people care about me. Some people never know that feeling. They go through life pondering the question, "If I die, I wonder who will come to my funeral?"

My friends gathered around me quickly and with a gusto I never knew was possible. Neighbors organized a plan to deliver meals to our family one day a week; coworkers took three days a week; and friends filled in the gaps. John and I didn't cook a meal for almost six months!

The night before I began chemotherapy, one of my friends threw a "chemotherapy shower." Fifteen women showed up for an evening of dinner, drinks, cards, and support.

Other friends would drop off surprises. I often came home from the hospital to find on my front porch packages containing gifts such as books, tapes, stationery, or rabbits to add to my collection of over three thousand.

One coworker, operating out of our New York office, sent me dozens of cards. I often received three or four a week, and he continued his ritual throughout my treatment.

My friends encouraged me to get back into life. So what if I didn't have any hair or the energy to go a full round of eighteen holes of golf? They were just glad to have me around, and I decided to enjoy every minute of every day.

I was touched by the number of men who called me once a week or once a month to check on my progress and see how I was doing. They didn't always know the "right" thing to say, and sometimes they sounded embarrassed when mentioning my illness, but I quickly assured them how much it meant to me that they cared enough to call.

Ironically, a dear friend had been diagnosed with breast cancer just two months before I was. It was comforting and encouraging to share our experiences, fears, and triumphs. Her positive attitude paved the way for my mental outlook. If she could do it, so could I!

I made a lot of new friends. People came from everywhere to offer words of advice, encouragement, and compassion. Don't ever be afraid to ask people for help when you need it. The love and support people want to give you in this situation can absolutely get you through each day.

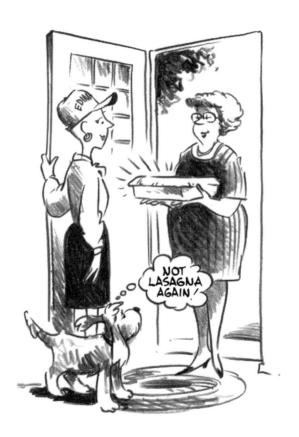

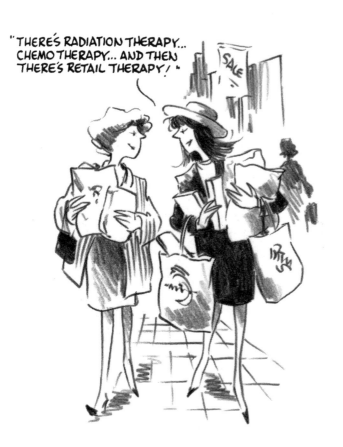

89

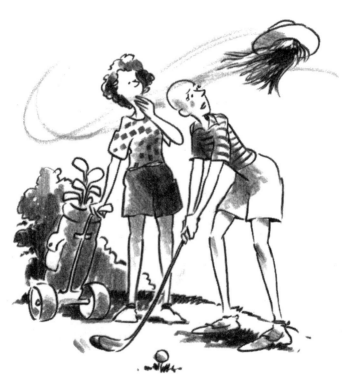

"DARN!... I KNEW I SHOULD HAVE WORN A CHIN STRAP."

91

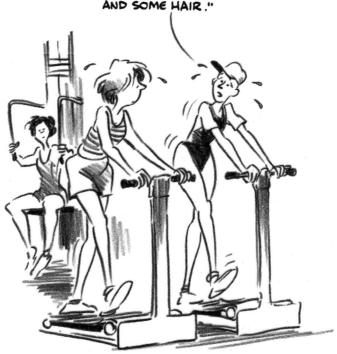

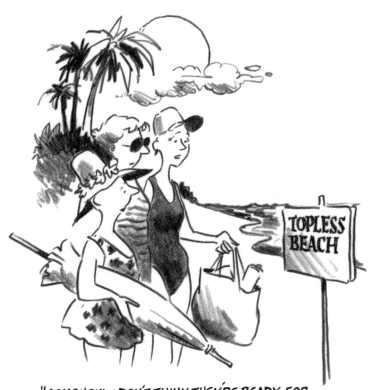

"SOMEHOW, I DON'T THINK THEY'RE READY FOR
'THE BABES OF BREAST CANCER'!"

93

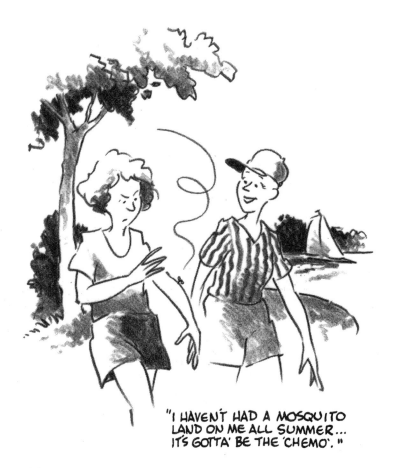

"I HAVEN'T HAD A MOSQUITO LAND ON ME ALL SUMMER... IT'S GOTTA' BE THE 'CHEMO'. "

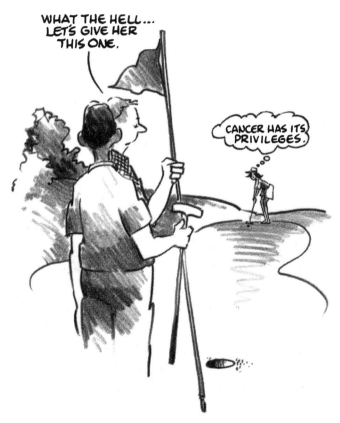

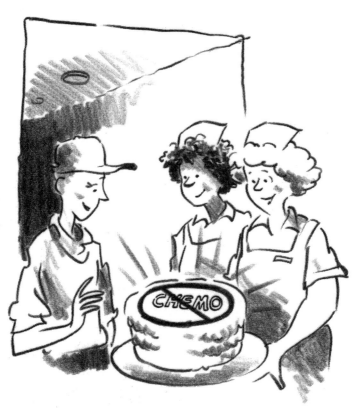

"GOOD LUCK, CHRIS...WE'LL MISS YOU."

Recovery: life after cancer

I've learned many things through my
experience with cancer—

that my life will never be the same; that there are people who give far more than the ordinary meaning of love and friendship, and that ultimately, if you look hard enough, something profoundly good can arise out of something bad.

Facing a diagnosis of cancer and the subsequent treatments can profoundly change the way we live the rest of our lives. We can wallow in self-pity with a "Why me?" attitude, or we can embrace the time we have left on this earth (cancer diagnosis or not), treasuring each and every moment, and treating each day as one full life.

When you feel discouraged, look all around you: at the beauty of the earth, the love of your family, and the support of your friends. The world is a better place because you are with them today.

If you are faced with a diagnosis of cancer or someone dear to you is going through the experience, give them a call or a hug or a smile.

And, oh yes, don't forget to laugh!

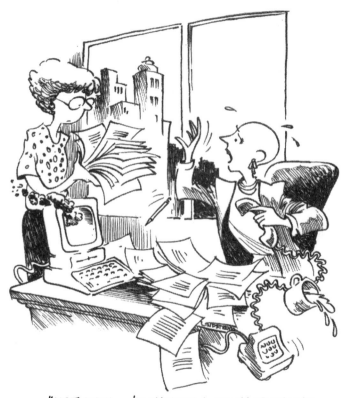

"NOT NOW... I'M HAVING A NO HAIR DAY!"

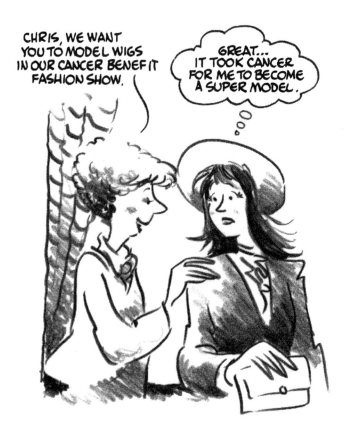

100

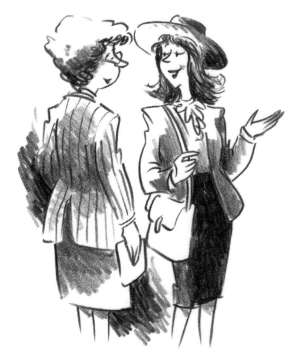

"WHY, THANKS FOR THE COMPLIMENT... BUT I OWE IT ALL
TO CHEMOTHERAPY. I'VE LOST TEN POUNDS... ANTIBIOTICS
HAVE DONE WONDERS FOR MY SKIN... AND MY HAIR
IS BORROWED FROM TWILA'S SALON."

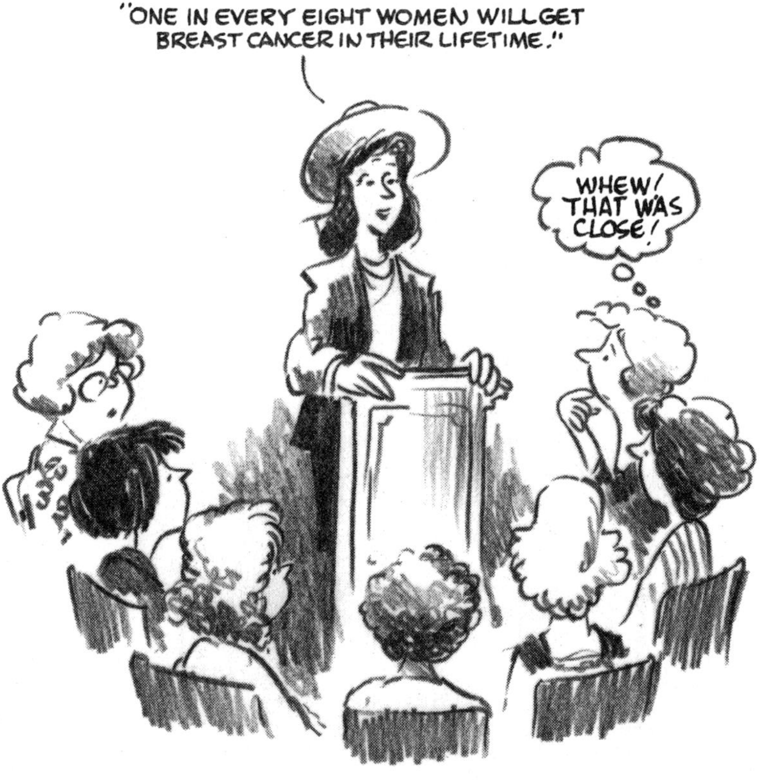
"ONE IN EVERY EIGHT WOMEN WILL GET BREAST CANCER IN THEIR LIFETIME."
WHEW! THAT WAS CLOSE!

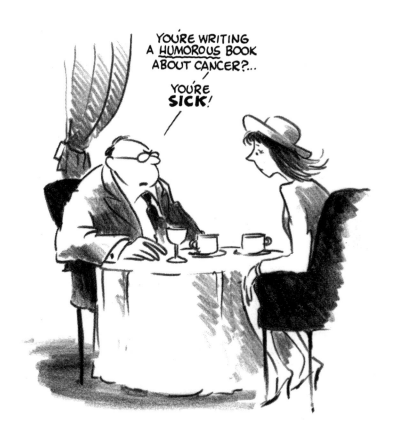

103

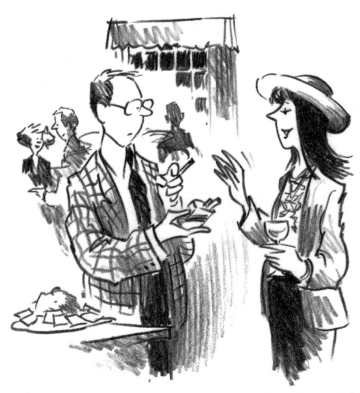

"GEE, NO THANKS...I ALREADY HAVE CANCER."

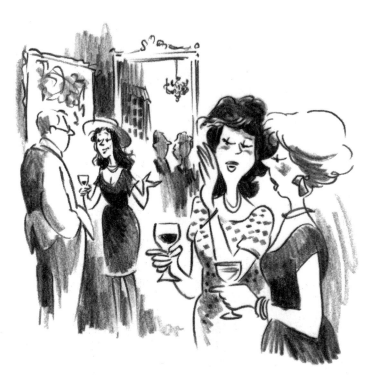

"I'M PRETTY SURE CHRIS IS WEARING A WIG... AND I'VE GOTTA' BELIEVE SHE HAD SOMETHING DONE TO HER BOOBS."

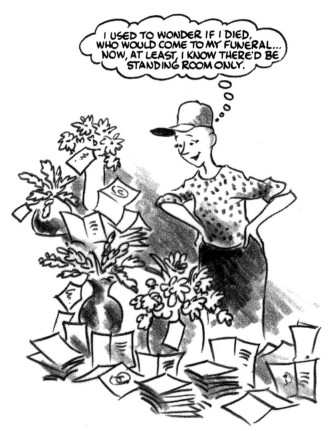

About the Author

Before her bout with breast cancer, Christine Clifford had definitely cracked the glass ceiling. At the age of forty, she was senior vice president for SPAR Marketing Services, an international information and merchandising services firm in Minneapolis, Minnesota.

As one of the top salespersons in the billion dollar service industry, Christine was responsible for accounts with Kmart, Toys "R" Us, Procter & Gamble, AT&T, Tyco Toys, and L'Oreal, among others.

A dynamic public speaker, she has lectured at events from the Garfield the Cat annual "Big Deal" to "Promoting in the 90s" and "How to Make Merchandising Work for You" seminars.

Chris is currently president and chief executive officer of The Cancer Club, a company designed to market helpful and humorous products for people who have cancer.

She lives with her husband, John, and sons, Tim and Brooks, and her dog, Sneakers, in Edina, Minnesota.

About the Illustrator

A native Minnesotan, Jack Lindstrom graduated with a bachelor of fine arts degree from the Minneapolis College of Art and Design and operates F.A.B. Artists, Inc., an art studio in Minneapolis.

He specializes in humorous illustration for various print media—books, periodicals, and newspapers. For the past ten years he has also collaborated with William Wells to produce a daily comic strip, "Executive Suite," for United Feature Syndicate.

Jack is married to his high school sweetheart, receives unsolicited advice from two grown children, and helps to spoil his three grandchildren whenever the opportunity presents itself.

The Cancer Club

The Cancer Club was formed in 1995 to produce and distribute humorous and helpful products for people with cancer. The Cancer Club is a fun company! Its charge is to lift the spirits of those whose lives have been touched by cancer: the patients, family, friends, caregivers, and survivors.

The Cancer Club has a full line of gift items for cancer patients including: books, tapes, custom jewelry, T-shirts, coffee mugs, notepads, etc. A quarterly newsletter is published with humorous and uplifting stories about people dealing with cancer.

Christine Clifford, founder and president of The Cancer Club, is available for seminars, workshops and 30–60 minute breakfast, lunch, or dinner speeches. Choose from lectures on health care, motivation, self empowerment, and recovery. Christine addresses conventions, associations, women's events, health care focused events, the corporate arena, public and private sector organizations.

For more information on The Cancer Club, call or write:

The Cancer Club
6533 Limerick Drive
Edina, MN 55439

(800) 586-9062
(612) 941-1229 fax

canclub@primenet.com
www.cancerclub.com